Survival Medicine
All You Need In Your First-Aid Kit + Medical Handbook

Table of content

Introduction..2

Chapter 1 – Why is Survival Medicine Important for You? 4

Benefits of Survival Medicine and Quick Medical Assistance 5

Chapter 2 – Setting Up Your First-Aid Kit...8

Basic Supplies You Need in Your First-Aid Kit 9

Some Precautions...12

Chapter 3 – Maintain Your First-Aid Kit..14

How to maintain your first-aid kit? 14

Keep your first-aid medical kit organized 16

Keep updating your first-aid kit 17

Chapter 4 – Necessary Things You Need in Your Medical Handbook............................19

Why do you need a medical handbook? 19

About what medical emergencies should my medical handbook offer me guidelines?...........20

FREE Bonus Reminder 27

Introduction

Accidents can happen anytime without former notice. This means you need to be prepared beforehand for emergency situations. Standing by an accident and not being able to do anything to help makes things more unpleasant. For such cases, you should be ready to give prompt and basic aid to the sufferer/s until the professionals jump in and take care of the situation. First aid is important because it helps controlling an emergency situation so that it doesn't get out of hand.

You should always have a first-aid kit with you and a medical handbook that has basic medical guidelines for you. In this book, you'll know what you need to do to make a complete first-aid kit that has everything you need in a survival situation or if you happen to witness an accident.

Time is very important in case of emergency situations. A person can literally die within seconds if he/she is not given basic medical attention. In this book, I'd teach you how to avoid that, how to save someone's life without losing a second.

For this book to help you fully, you'd need a lot of courage. Emergencies and accidents are not for the faint-hearted people. The sight of blood, suffering, injuries and even simple wounds can shake you if you are not brave enough. So first of all, you'd have to be brave for someone else so that he/she can be saved. It'd not be difficult if you really think about the difference you'd be making in somebody else's life. You could be saving lives so stand up and be brave for humanity.

This book would help you understand why first-aid is important and how can you set up your own first aid kit that has everything you need for every possible emergency.

Chapter 1 – Why is Survival Medicine Important for You?

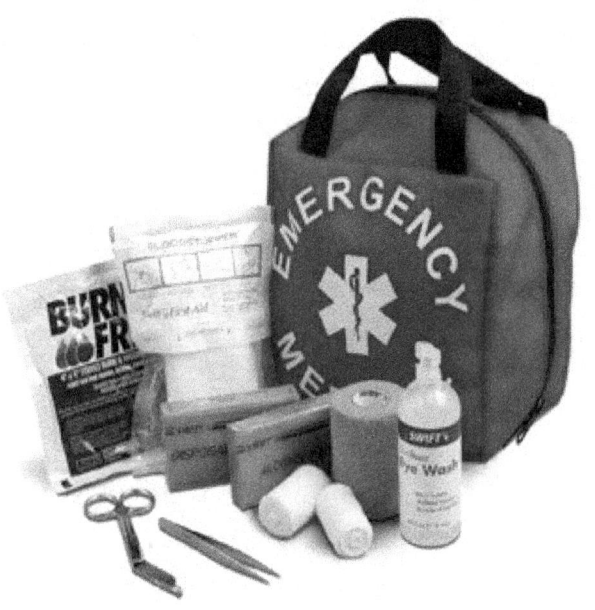

First things first! Why is survival medicine important when you have doctors and paramedics to help? The answer is simple. Suppose you're driving back home and on your way back you witness two cars colliding each other. What would you do? You'd stop your car and you'll call 911 in an instant. Now, it's obvious that it would take time for 911 to reach the site of an accident. What would you do until then? Wait? No, because, there are a bunch of people bleeding immensely. They might be in a critical condition situation. Now waiting for the professionals to come and handle the situation that is getting worse with every passing second, would not be a wise decision on your end. How would you feel if you had a first aid kit and knowledge of survival medicine to help you alleviate the suffering of the people in distress? This is why survival medicine is really important, for situations like these.

Survival medicine is important because only then you'd be able to give initial assistance to someone who's injured or ill. Initial assistant is just to control a deteriorating situation so that it doesn't get out of hand until the professionals arrive. First-aid can be given by a layperson with some basic equipment and medicine in their first-aid kit. And if you don't have that, you'd just be a bystander who'd see the situation getting worse and would not be able to do anything about it.

Benefits of Survival Medicine and Quick Medical Assistance

Let's have a look at some of the benefits of survival medicine and quick medical assistance,

- **Your family and home would be safe:** The biggest benefit of learning first aid and quick medical assistance is that your home would be a safe place. How? You'd be more and more cautious about things and if there's an accident, you'd be able to take things under your control and alleviate your family member's suffering until the doctors reach you.

- **Your workplace would be safer:** You know how to give quick medical assistance in times of need; this means your workplace would feel a lot safer with you. If your colleague is having a seizure or is physically hurt somehow, you'd be able to help him/her.

- **You can save lives:** If you know how to give instant medical assistance to a person in distress, you are a life saver. You can save a lot of lives if a natural disaster strikes down or if there's a road accident on your way home.

- **It can reduce recovery time:** Wounds and injuries take a lot of time to heal if they're left open and unattended for a long period of time and this is very common when someone is injured in a road accident and the paramedics are on their way. If you are there at the time of a road accident and you know how to stop the wound from getting infected and you have a first-aid medical of your own too, it would help reduce the recovery time of the wound or injury.

- **You could help the suffering person in an emergency or distress:** If you're there when a person suddenly gets an asthma attack, or swallows something poisonous, or gets ill or if a natural disaster occurs, you'd not just be a bystander like most of the people standing there. You'd be able to help not only the suffering party but you'd also be able to stop things from getting worse even for the paramedics and doctors.

- **You could assist the suffering party in the right way:** This is very important that the person suffering gets the right treatment. If you're not knowledgeable about how to give the right medical assistance to the person suffering, you might make things worse to an extent that the even professionals won't be able to handle it. Survival medicine in first-aid ensures that you know exactly what you're doing and you're confident about it.

- **You could help yourself:** Your first-aid and survival medicine knowledge is not just helpful to other people in distress; you could also make use of this knowledge to help yourself too.

Accidents keep happening and we don't know when or where we would have to face an emergency situation. To be able to tackle situations like these, it is important that you have first-aid knowledge. Fatalities often are a result of lack of instant medical treatment. Survival medicine and first-aid would ensure that quick medical assistance is given to not only stop the matters from getting out of our hands but also to save lives. And keeping a first-aid kit and a medical handbook with you always would help you tackle sudden emergencies.

Chapter 2 – Setting Up Your First-Aid Kit

Knowledge of survival medicine and first-aid alone is of no use if you don't have the necessary equipment and medicines to help you carry out the required treatments. For example, if you find an injured person bleeding out on the road and you know how to take care of his wounds and how to bandage him, what medicines to use but you don't have those medicines with you and it would take some time until help arrives and there's no pharmacy nearby either. What good would your knowledge of survival medicine be if you can't help someone in distress? For cases such as these, what you need is a first-aid kit with you.

Carrying a well-equipped first-aid kit with you all the time would help you cope with sudden natural disasters, road-side accidents, sudden illness, injuries and wounds etc. There are many drugstores and pharmacies where you could get your hands on a good first-aid kit. But I suggest that you assemble a first-aid kit of your own. In this chapter, you'd know what necessary medicines and equipment you should have to complete your own first-aid kit.

Here's a list of supplies and medicines and other necessary stuff that are essential for a complete and well-stocked first-aid kit.

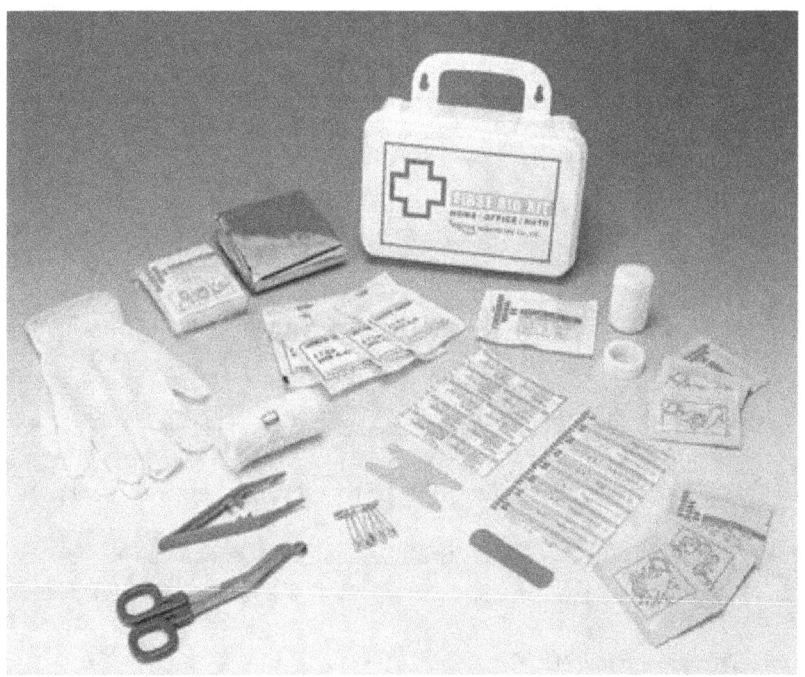

Basic Supplies You Need in Your First-Aid Kit

First, you'd need to get some basic supplies for your first-aid kit. Here's a list of these supplies,

- A water bottle - To drink or clean wounds or injuries

- Disposable non-latex examination gloves, several pairs - To prevent bacteria and germs from hands to transfer to a wound or injury

- Adhesive tape - To hold splints or dressing together

- Duct tape

- Cotton balls and cotton buds - To apply ointments or other solutions to wounds or injuries

- Absorbent cotton rolls - To use as a padding for a splint

- Eye pads

- Elastic wrap bandages

- Bandage strips (Different sizes) - To use on minor or major cuts and abrasions

- Butterfly bandages - To hold the cuts together to let them heal

- Roller gauzes (Different sizes) - To support sprained muscles or sore parts

- Sterile gauze pads - To control bleeding or secretions and prevent the injury or wound from festering

- Triangular bandages - To support a broken limb

- A lubricant (Petroleum jelly)

- Aluminum finger splint

- Instant cold packs - For contusions or bruises

- Plastic bags (Different sizes)

- Safety pins (Different sizes)

- Scissors

- Tweezers

- Hand sanitizer - To keep your hands germs and bacteria free

- Thermometer

- Suction device (Turkey baster)

- Breathing barrier

- Syringes

- Medicine cups or spoons

- Face and dust masks - To protect against dust, germs or allergens

- A First-aid manual

Next, you'd need to get the following medications for your first-aid kit,

- Eyewash solution

- Antibiotic ointment - To prevent minor wounds or injuries from getting infected

- Calamine lotion - To relieve pain and prevent itching caused by poison, insect bites, burns or rashes

- Antacids - To reduce symptoms of Acid Reflux

- Antiseptic solution or ointment - To clean wounds or injuries

- Aloe vera gel - to heal wounds or skin inflammation

- Anti-diarrhea medication

- Laxative - To increase bowel movements

- Antihistamine, such as diphenhydramine - For allergic reactions

- Pain relievers, (Tylenol, Advil, Ibuprofen, Aspirins etc) - Aspirin is not for children

- Hydrocortisone cream - To reduce chemical reactions on the skin

- Cough and cold medications

In the case of emergencies, you should be all set. Below is a list of items you would need in emergencies,

- A list of emergency phone numbers like emergency road service providers, poison helpline etc

- A small flashlight that is water resistant

- Extra batteries

- Waterproof writing equipment and notepads

- Waterproof matches

- A phone with a solar charger

- Insect repellents

- Sunscreen

The lists given above contain everything that you would need in times of emergencies. If you get everything from the list, you'd be able to handle any problem you come across.

Some Precautions

Now that you have all that you need in your first-aid kit, here are some of the precautions you have to make sure that you'd take care of,

- Keep your first-aid kit away from the reach of your children.

- Always take your first-aid kit with you, wherever you go. Even to work.

- Always read the instructions on the medication before you take them.

- Keep a special check on the expiry dates of the medications you have in your first-aid kit. Make sure you've disposed of the medicines that have expired and replaced them with fresh ones.

- Aspirins are not for children. Don't give it to them.

- Don't buy medicines that have cuts or tears on their packs.

- Make sure you know all about the medicines you have in your first-aid kit.

- Consider participating in a first-aid course provided by different organizations.

- Teach your children a little about first-aid too, depending on their age.

If you have everything mentioned in this chapter, fear not, you'd be able to cope almost all sorts of emergency situations that require instant medical attention. Keep this first-aid kit with you everywhere you go and prove yourself useful to the people in distress.

Chapter 3 – Maintain Your First-Aid Kit

You've completed your medical first aid-kit. It's good news that you've not gotten any chance to use it because that means, you have not encountered an emergency or a natural disaster or a road accident etc. But it doesn't mean you can leave your first-aid kid unattended. Once you've set up your first-aid kit, it doesn't mean, your job has finished and that this was all to it. No. It's a continuous job. You cannot just leave your first-aid kit in some corner of your room. You'd have to keep a check on it. You'd have to see if the medications have expired. If yes, you'd have to dispose of them immediately. It is a very common mistake that we make with everything. We buy something and we think that this is it and there's nothing more you should do. That's not true. Let's say, for example, you've bought a car, would leave it like that in the garage forever even if you're using it regularly? No. you won't, because, that way it would stop working eventually. Why? Because, you have done nothing to take care of it! You have never checked if your car needed maintenance. Yes! Just like your car and everything else, you'd need to maintain your first-aid kit too. Here's how you can do that.

How to maintain your first-aid kit?

After you've gotten all the supplies and medications for your first-aid kit, you'd need to store them in some place safe and where they are not open to getting contaminated. This is very important that you make sure your first-aid kit is somewhere, 1) Safe and clean and 2) you can access it anytime you want.

Some tips on maintaining your first-aid kit,

- **Select the right container:** This is the first thing you should be doing. Selecting the right container for your supplies and medicines. Get a container that is water resistant. This is important because it can happen that you have to work in the rain. Select a container that is lightweight and durable. There are many options in the market that you can choose from.

- **Keep the supplies in an order:** To maintain your first-aid kit as efficiently as possible, you'd have to make sure you do that in an orderly manner. Whether your first-aid kit is a box or a bag, you should make sure that everything is kept in an orderly fashion. Why? Because there are certain liquids and solutions that can spill in your kit damaging other supplies too which means you'd not be able to use almost anything from your first-aid kit. So order is the first step to maintaining your first-aid kit.

- **Keep the liquids and fluids tight shut** - To avoid any spills, you have to make sure all the solutions and liquids in your first-aid kit are tightly shut. You don't have to be an expert to understand that liquid spill can damage other supplies too. And then you'd have to unpack and repack your whole first-aid medical kit again.

- **Keep your first-aid medical kit at room temperature** - Wherever you want to keep your first-aid kit, make sure the temperature is not very high and not very low. Because there are medicines in your first-aid kit that require to be kept at room temperature to keep them from damaging.

Keep your first-aid medical kit organized

Why do you want to do this? Because there are just so many things stuffed in your first-aid kid that in times of need, you might want something, let's say you want the bandages. Where are the bandages? They might be somewhere beneath all the pile of other bandages, cotton balls and gauzes. A lot of time would be wasted in finding just the bandages. What would happen when you'd need to find other tablets and medications? To save time and lives, it is mighty important that you keep your first-aid kit in an organized way. How can you do that? You can divide all the supplies and medicines into a few categories. The categories can be,

1. Equipment to treat wounds and injuries

2. Prescription medication

3. Ointments and solutions

4. Other supplies

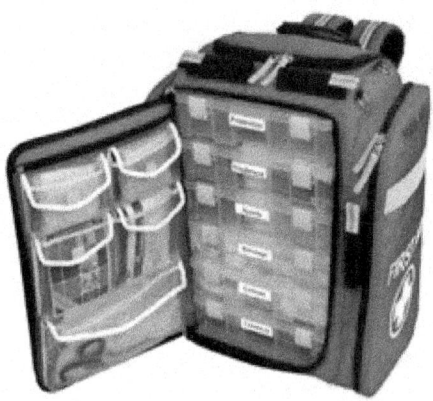

Now keeping in mind these categories, you'd separate all the stuff in four parts. And then you can keep them together in separate sections of your first-aid kit. This way you'd be able to find the right thing in the right section without wasting any time in finding that thing.

Keep updating your first-aid kit

Now that your first-aid kit is all set and you know how to keep it maintained and you are ready to serve humanity in the times of natural disasters or accidents or any such emergencies. But your work doesn't stop here. Like I've said before, your medical kit would need to be checked every now and then. You wouldn't want to end up using expired medication by mistake on the suffering party and make things much, much worse.

Now this is the thing I'll put a lot of emphasis on. This is very important that you keep checking your first-aid kit if it needs anything new, if the medicines and other supplies can still be used or have they expired? Check your kit for any used up supplies. Do that often if you need to use your first-aid kit very often.

It would be really helpful if you keep a checklist of all the items in your first-aid kit with your all the time. With this, you can keep a track of everything that is used up or expired or need replacing. If you don't know what you're doing, it would be really difficult for you to maintain your first-aid kit. But if you do it systematically and in an orderly fasion, one thing at a time, it would be really easy.

Yes. It is true that keeping a first-aid medical kit is not a fun job but nobody does it for fun. It's done to serve humanity and help people out when they need it. Keeping a first-aid medical kit can cost you a lot. It doesn't matter if you've bought a ready-made first-aid medical kit or you've built yourself one, it is always going to cost you. You'd always have to keep checking it and buy new supplies that have either expired or finished up. But this shouldn't stop you from getting a first-aid medical kit because this is something that you don't do for money but for the sake of a good cause. Plus, if ever you need to use your first-aid medical kit, you'd realize that it was worth every penny that you've spent setting it up and maintaining it.

Chapter 4 – Necessary Things You Need in Your Medical Handbook

In the previous chapters you have learned how to set up a first-aid medical kit for yourself and how to maintain that medical kit in order to keep it working for you. Now that you have learnt how to set up a first-aid medical kit and how to take care of it in the best way possible, what should you need more to be able to do everything there is to help the suffering party? A complete medical handbook of course!

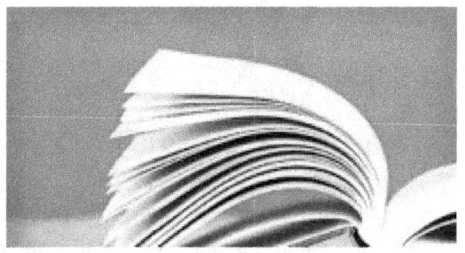

Why do you need a medical handbook?

The answer to this question is really simple. If you face an emergency situation that you have no knowledge about, a medical handbook would help you handle it. A medical handbook would teach you simple procedures like how to cover a wound and prevent it from getting infected, or how to give a CPR, or how to handle deep cuts and wounds etc.

Now the question that next comes to mind is what kind of a medical handbook should you keep with you always? Obviously, there are many medical handbooks available in the market that cover all kinds of medical topics. Which one should you choose for your guidance? Below are some points that you should keep in mind before you buy a medical handbook to keep with your first-aid kit.

- Buy a basic book that some basic stuff about quick medical treatment and first-aid.

- Don't buy a book that has a lot of pro stuff written in it.

- Look for a medical handbook that has step by step guidelines as well as pictures to explain different medical treatments and situations to you.

- Buy a book that is easy to understand. A book that a layperson can keep for his/her guidance.

- Buy a book that would teach you how to handle emergency situations in simple and easy steps.

- This handbook should contain guidelines about simple quick medical treatments like CPR, stroke treatment etc.

About what medical emergencies should my medical handbook offer me guidelines?

The answer to this question is a difficult one because there are so many different medical situations that you may have to face all of a sudden and to say how can you be prepared for all of them, would not be rational. But there are some general and main medical assistance procedures that come on handy in almost all kinds of emergencies. Be it a natural disaster or a road accident or an animal bite. Let's dig deeply into the above points and see what treatments and medical guidelines your medical handbook should offer you that can prove helpful in almost all emergency situations.

- **Short breathing** - Your medical handbook should be able to guide you on how to cope with a situation in which the victim is having difficulties breathing.

- **Choking** - Your medical handbook should guide you on how to help someone who's choking. The handbook should explain the symptoms of choking and how to treat it.

- **Nosebleed** - This is is a common medical situation. Your medical handbook should be able to guide you on causes of nosebleed and how to treat them instantly.

- **Broken bones** - Before you get the victim to a doctor or a doctor comes to him/her, you should be able to give some quick medical assistance to the suffering person so that matters don't get out of your hands by the time the doctor arrives. This should all be explained in easy term in your medical handbook.

- **Avoid infections** - Injuries and wounds are really sensitive areas. They are a way for the bacterias and germs to get into the body easily. If they remain open for a long period of time and are not cleaned up, they may get infected which would make the matters worse than they were before. Your medical handbook should guide you on how to clean minor or major wounds and how to prevent them from getting infected.

- **Bruises and contusions** - Bruises and contusions are common and they must be taken care of. Your medical handbook should tell you how to treat different bruises and contusions on a human body.

- **Alleviate pain** - When the sufferer is in pain, you'd first need to lessen his suffering by giving him pain relievers. There should be enough information on the use and dose of pain killers in your medical handbook.

- **Treat allergies** - Your medical handbook should explain how to treat different kinds of allergies and the causes behind them.

- **Treat bites, poisons and stings** - Getting bit by a stray dog, or a snake or a wasp's sting is something not very rare. Your medical handbook should tell you how to treat different bites and stings before you take the victim to the doctor.

- **Heat stroke** - This is something that is common in places that are hot and humid. Your medical handbook should contain information and guidelines on how to treat heat stroke.

- **Vomiting and nausea** - Get a medical handbook that has guidelines about treating vomiting and nausea in case of emergencies.

- **Seizures** - A complete medical handbook should teach the reader on how to handle a person who is having different kinds of seizures. How to help him until the professionals arrive.

- **High fever** - If someone's suffering from a high fever, you should have a medical handbook that has guidelines on how to keep the fever from going up and maintain body temperature until the doctors come to the rescue.

- **Frostnip** - It is a mild freezing cold wound and your medical handbook should have information on the symptoms and how to treat it.

- **Frostbite** - Make sure that you've bought a handbook that can teach you how to treat frostbite and what are the causes and the symptoms.

- **Hypothermia** - Temperature drops and severe cold can cause the human body to lose its temperature. Make sure that you have selected a medical handbook that has enough information on how to identify the symptoms of hypothermia and how to treat it.

- **Gas inhalation** - If someone's inhaled a dangerous gas, you should know what to do about it. Buy a medical handbook that can help you recognize what kind of gas the victim has inhaled and how it can be treated.

- **Use of basic medical equipment in your first-aid kit** - Your medical handbook should cover all there is about different basic medical equipment that one keeps in a first-aid box.

This was a more specific list of things you should have in your medical handbook that you've bought. Make sure your medical handbook provides assistance to the above problems because they are the most common problems you'll be facing in the times of distress. You'd need the medical handbook to help you when you're confused and not sure about what to do with a certain kind of problem. Finding the best medical handbook that would help you handle almost all kinds of emergency situations is not an easy job. So take your time and deeply search for the best medical handbook out there. Don't make haste. Scan and skim through different medical handbooks before you finally decide on buying the right one. Because you don't want to face an emergency and realize that there is nothing about it in the medical handbook that you have selected. The above list should help you and if you think of anything else that should also be on this list, be open to look for that in your medical handbook too. Otherwise, the above list covers almost everything you'd want in a complete medical handbook.

Conclusion

To conclude this book, I'll say that everyone should set up a first-aid kit and get a medical handbook that contains everything there is to quick medical assistance and first-air. If you've read this book and understood everything, you'd know that first-aid knowledge is really important in times of distress. You could be saving lives and alleviating pain. It's a big task for a layperson.

The best thing about first-aid is that you don't have to be a professional to do this. All you need is some basic medical knowledge (take a first-aid course) and the desire to help humanity to do that if you really wants to do something and make a difference.

With a first-aid kit of your own, you'd not look at other people doe help and you'd certainly not be a helpless spectator or a sad bystander at the site of an emergency or when a natural catastrophe struck down. You'd be someone who could save the day, a superhero, and a person who helped saved lives, someone who really matters.

If you're going to get started with your first-aid kit, good luck. Make sure you have everything in your box and that you take it with you everywhere you go for as I've mentioned earlier, what good would your first-aid kit be if you forget it at home and don't have it when you need it on the road or a trip to some other city.

Also be cautious about maintaining your first-aid kit, keeping in check the expiry dates of all the medications and ointments and different medical solutions. Make sure you buy medicines, bandages, cotton buds etc that have used up. Make a list of all the equipment of your first-aid kit and keep a check on everything that you need to buy because either it's used up or has expired. Because you'd not want to feel helpless if you need a certain medication in an emergency situation but when you check the bottle, it's empty.

Keep the kit safe and away from the reach of your children and make sure it has everything you need, especially when you're leaving your home. Keep it with you every time you leave home. Good luck serving humanity!

FREE Bonus Reminder

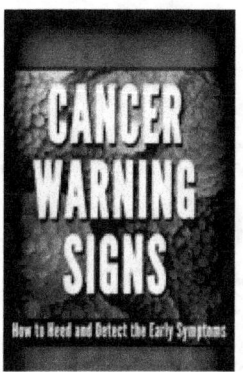

If you have not grabbed it yet, please go ahead and download your special bonus report *"DIY Projects. 13 Useful & Easy To Make DIY Projects To Save Money & Improve Your Home!"*
Simply Click the Button Below

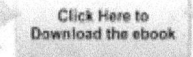

OR **Go to This Page**
http://healthylivingpeople.com/free/

BONUS #2: More Free & Discounted Books
Do you want to receive more Free & Discounted Books?

We have a mailing list where we send out our new Books when they go free or with a discount on Kindle. Click on the link below to sign up for Free & Discount Book Promotions.

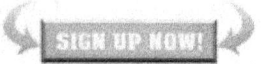

www.ingramcontent.com/pod-product-compliance
Lightning Source LLC
Chambersburg PA
CBHW071203220526
45468CB00003B/1148